Meal Prep

154 Delicious, Quick, and Low-Carb Recipe Cookbook For Weight Loss And Healthy Living

Table of Contents

Introduction

I would like to thank you and congratulate you for purchasing the book, *Meal Prep: 147 Delicious, Easy and Wholesome Recipes for Weight Loss and Healthy Living.*

This book contains proven steps and strategies on how to start meal prepping. If you are trying to get healthy or lose some weight, the most common drawback is to eat and drink mindlessly. So even if strict calorie counting and meal planning are observed, unplanned snacks and beverages could ruin your diet. This is why meal prepping is very important.

This book contains basic information on how to prepare healthy and energy-boosting meals that are easy to make and prepare, and can be done at the least possible amount of time.

This book also provides a good number of meal prep recipes that you can follow on a day to day basis so you won't eat or drink absentmindedly. The recipes you will find here are customized to encourage the body to organically help you become healthy and lose weight given a short span of time.

Thanks again for purchasing this book! I hope you enjoy it!

Chapter 1
Breakfast Meal Prep Ideas

Almond-Coconut Bread

Ingredients:

- coconut oil for greasing loaf tin

- 4 tablespoons coconut flour

- 4 cups almond flour

- 1 teaspoon baking soda

- ½ cup flaxseed meal

- ½ teaspoon sea salt

- 2 tablespoons coconut vinegar

- 10 large eggs, whisked

Directions:

1. Preheat the oven to 350°F.

2. Lightly grease loaf tin. Mix coconut flour, almond flour, baking soda, flaxseed meal, and salt. Make a well in the center and pour coconut vinegar and eggs. Mix well until just combined. Pour batter into loaf tin.

3. Bake for 35 minutes or until toothpick inserted in center comes out clean. Remove pan from oven. Allow cake to cool completely. Slice and serve plain or toasted.

Oats with Berries and Walnuts

Ingredients:

For the oats

- 1 cup water

- 1 cup almond milk

- 1 cup steel-cut oat

- Dash of nutmeg powder

- Drop of vanilla extract

Walnut-berry sauce

- ½ cup raw walnut, chopped

- ½ cup water

- ¼ cup fresh or frozen raspberries

- ¼ cup fresh or frozen blueberries

- ¼ cup fresh or frozen cranberries

- ¼ cup fresh or frozen strawberries

- 1 Tbsp. raisins

- 1 tsp. stevia

- 1 tsp. lemon juice, freshly squeezed

Directions:

1. For the oats, except for vanilla extract, pour all ingredients in a sauce pan set over medium heat. Let this come to a soft boil.

2. Immediately turn down heat to lowest setting. Partially put lid on. Let oats cook for 15 to 20 minutes, stirring often. Oats should be runny. Add more water, if needed.

3. Remove sauce pan from heat. Add in vanilla extract. Stir. Let oats cool slightly, uncovered.

4. For the walnut-berry sauce, toast walnuts in skillet set over medium heat. Shake skillet often. Walnuts are done when these become aromatic and slightly deeper in color. Set aside.

5. Add remaining ingredients of walnut-berry sauce except for stevia and lemon juice, in another sauce pan.

6. Let this come to a full boil while stirring often. Mash berries lightly to release more flavor.

7. Cook until sauce is reduced and thickened, about 3 to 5 minutes. Stir in stevia and lemon juice.

8. To serve, ladle ½ cup of cooked oats into a small bowl. Drizzle in berry sauce on top.

9. Sprinkle a pinch of toasted walnuts on top. Serve immediately.

Cashew Carrots Muffin

Ingredients:

- 1½ cups whole wheat pastry flour
- 2 teaspoons baking soda
- 4 large carrots, shredded
- 2 servings flax eggs
- ½ cup steel-cut oats
- ½ cup brown sugar
- ¼ cup coconut oil
- 1 teaspoon vanilla extract
- ¼ cup cashew nuts, chopped

Directions:

1. Preheat oven to 375°F.
2. Place paper liners into muffin tins. Combine pastry flour, baking soda, carrots, flax eggs, oats, and brown sugar, oil, vanilla extract, and cashew nuts. Do not over mix.
3. Spoon batter into muffin depressions.
4. Bake for 20 minutes or until toothpick inserted in center comes out clean. Remove from oven. Allow to cool before serving.

Oats with Avocadoes and Apples

Ingredients:

- ½ cup milk

- ¼ cup steel-cut oats

- 2 avocadoes, chopped

- 1 apple, chopped

- 1 carrots, chopped

Directions:

1. In a microwave-safe bowl, mix milk, oats, avocadoes, apples, and carrots. Stir well.

2. Microwave on highest setting for 15 seconds or before milk bubbles out of the bowl.

3. Remove bowl from the microwave. Allow to cool.

4. Sprinkle almond nuts on top. Serve.

Plantain Crisps

Ingredients:

- 8 ripe plantains, peeled, quartered lengthwise

- olive oil for drizzling

- Dash of Spanish paprika

- Pinch of sea salt

Directions:

1. Preheat the oven to 250°F. Line a baking sheet with aluminum foil.

2. Layer plantains on baking sheets with spaces in between pieces. Drizzle in oil. Season with paprika and salt. Bake for 1 hours.

3. Cool completely to room temperature. Serve.

Mock Pancakes

Ingredients:

- 1 egg

- 1 cup ricotta cheese

- 1 tsp. cinnamon

- 2 tbsp. honey, add more if needed

Directions:

1. Using a blender, put together egg, honey, cinnamon, and ricotta cheese. Process until all ingredients are well combined.

2. Pour an equal amount of the blended mixture into the pan. Cook each pancake for 4 minutes on both sides. Serve.

Mushrooms Bruschetta on Hummus

Ingredients:

- 1 slice toasted Coriander Bread

- ½ tablespoon Hummus

- ¼ teaspoon coriander, minced

- ½ cup canned straw mushrooms, halved

- ½ tablespoon cashew cheese

- Pinch of kosher salt

- Pinch of white pepper

Directions:

1. In a bowl, combine hummus, coriander, straw mushrooms, and cashew cheese. Season with salt and pepper.

2. Spread on top of bread. Heat in a toaster oven. Serve.

Oats with Berries and Avocadoes

Ingredients:

- ½ cup milk

- ¼ cup steel-cut oats

- ¼ cup raspberries

- ½ avocado, diced into bite-sized pieces

- ½ teaspoon almond nuts, lightly roasted

Directions:

1. In a microwave-safe bowl, mix milk, oats, raspberries and avocado. Stir well.

2. Microwave on highest setting for 15 seconds or before milk bubbles out of the bowl.

3. Remove bowl from the microwave. Allow to cool.

4. Sprinkle almond nuts on top. Serve.

Mexican Frittata with Wheat Belly Taco Seasoning

Ingredients:

- ½ cup almond milk

- 5 large eggs

- ¼ cup onions, chopped

- ¼ cup green bell pepper, chopped

- ¾ cup parmesan cheese

- 2 tablespoons Wheat Belly Taco Seasoning – refer to recipe below

- Pinch of salt

- Pinch of pepper

- 1 cup of salsa

Directions:

1. Preheat the oven to 400 F.

2. Using a large bowl, combine almond milk, eggs, onion, green bell pepper, cheese, and taco seasoning. Season with salt, and pepper. Whisk until all ingredients are well combined.

3. Transfer the mixture in a baking dish. Bake for 20 minutes.

4. Cut and serve. Top with salsa.

Wheat Belly Taco Seasoning

Ingredients:

- 1 ½ teaspoons garlic powder

- 1 ½ teaspoons onion powder

- 1 teaspoon ground cumin

- 1 teaspoon ground red pepper

- 1 teaspoon oregano, dried

- 1 ½ teaspoons paprika

- 2 tablespoons chili powder

Directions:

1. In a bowl, combine garlic powder, onion powder, cumin, ground red pepper, oregano, paprika, and chili powder. Mix well.

2. Store in an airtight container. Use as needed.

Crostini with Basil and Sun-Dried Tomatoes

Ingredients:

- 2 slices wheat bread, toasted

- 2 large garlic cloves, peeled

- ⅛ teaspoon avocado oil

For the Toppings:

- 1 fresh tomato, diced

- 2 pieces sun-dried tomatoes in oil, julienned

- 3 fresh basil leaves, julienned

- Pinch of sea salt

- Pinch of white pepper

Directions:

1. Preheat the oven toaster. Rub garlic cloves on the toasted bread. Set aside.

2. Top with sun-dried tomatoes, fresh tomatoes, and basil. In a small bowl, combine chicken, onion, avocado, celery rib, cashew nuts, salt and pepper. Adjust seasoning.

3. Spread on bread slices. Place in the oven toaster to warm through. Garnish with chives. Serve.

Mushroom Bruschetta

Ingredients:

- 1 slice whole wheat bread

- 1 tablespoon basil-cashew pesto sauce

- 1 teaspoon olive oil

- 1 large porcini mushroom, thinly sliced

- 1 garlic clove, minced

- 1 teaspoon parsley, minced

- 1 tablespoon balsamic vinegar

- Pinch of salt

- 1 teaspoon palm sugar

Directions:

1. Spread basil-cashew pesto sauce on one side of the bread. Set aside.

2. Meanwhile, in a skillet over medium heat, saute mushrooms. Add garlic, parsley, balsamic vinegar, salt, and sugar. Stir well.

3. Let it simmer for 5 minutes. Remove from heat.

4. Spoon mixture ad spread on top of the bread. Serve.

Grilled Plantains with Coconut Flakes

Ingredients:

- Coconut butter for greasing

- 8 ripe plantains, peeled, quartered lengthwise

- ¼ cup almond flakes, toasted

- ¼ cup coconut flakes, toasted

Directions:

1. Preheat electric grill.

2. Grease plantain slivers with coconut butter.

3. Grill until brown on both sides. Remove from heat. Drizzle in coconut flakes and almond.

Oatmeal Muffins

Ingredients:

- 1½ cups whole wheat pastry flour

- 1 teaspoon baking powder

- 1 teaspoon baking soda

- ½ cup steel cut oats

- 2 servings flax eggs

- 1¼ cups coconut milk

- ¼ cup coconut oil

- ¼ cup pure maple syrup

- 1 teaspoon vanilla extract

- ½ teaspoon kosher salt

Directions:

1. Preheat oven to 375°F.

2. Place paper liners into muffin tins. Combine flour, baking powder, baking soda, and oats. In another bowl, combine flax eggs, coconut milk, coconut oil, maple syrup, vanilla extract, and salt. Stir until well combined.

3. Spoon batter into muffin depressions.

4. Bake for 25 minutes or until toothpick comes out clean. Remove from oven. Cool muffins before serving.

Oats with Apple and Berries

Ingredients:

- ½ cup milk

- ¼ cup steel-cut oats

- ¼ cup blueberries

- ½ apple, diced into bite-sized pieces

- ½ teaspoon cashew nuts, lightly roasted

Directions:

1. In a microwave-safe bowl, mix milk, oats, blueberries, and apple. Stir well.

2. Microwave on highest setting for 15 seconds or before milk bubbles out of the bowl.

3. Remove bowl from the microwave. Allow to cool.

4. Sprinkle cashew nuts on top. Serve.

Mock Cream Cheese Pancake

Ingredients:

- 2 cups cream cheese

- ½ teaspoon cinnamon

- 2 eggs

- 1 pack Stevia

Directions:

1. Put eggs, cream cheese, Stevia, and cinnamon in a blender. Process until all ingredients are well-combined.

2. Pour an equal amount of the blended mixture in a greased pan. Cook for 4 minutes on both sides. Repeat with the rest of the batter. Serve.

Olive Oil and Sesame Asparagus

Ingredients:

- ½ cup water

- 2 cups asparagus, sliced

- ½ tablespoon olive oil, add more for drizzling

- 1/8 teaspoon red pepper flakes, crushed

- ½ tablespoon light soy sauce, gluten-free

- ½ teaspoon sesame seeds

Directions:

1. In a large skillet, bring water to a boil.

2. Add in asparagus. Allow to boil for 2 minutes. Reduce the heat and cook for another 5 minutes. Drain asparagus place in a plate. Set aside.

3. Meanwhile, heat the olive oil. Tip in asparagus, red pepper flakes, and soy sauce. Saute for 3 minutes.

4. Remove from heat. Drizzle in more olive oil and sprinkle sesame seeds before serving.

Cashew Cheese

Ingredients:

- 1 cup raw cashew nuts, soaked in water overnight

- 1 teaspoon lemon juice, fresh squeezed, pips removed

- ⅛ teaspoon sea salt

- 2 cups water, filtered

Directions:

1. In a food processor, combine lemon juice, almonds, and salt. Pour water and process until smooth.

2. Drape cheesecloth into fine-meshed. Pour in mixture to drain. Tie cheesecloth into a knot. Gently squeeze out liquids. Set aside for 1 day.

3. Place cheese in the fridge for 1 hour to set. Remove cheesecloth. Slice cheese.

Pecan Cheese

Ingredients:

- 1 cup raw pecan nuts, soaked in water overnight

- 1 teaspoon lemon juice, fresh squeezed

- ⅛ teaspoon sea salt

- 2 cups water, filtered

- 1 fresh apricot, diced for garnish

Directions:

1. In a food processor, combine lemon juice, almonds, and salt. Pour water and process until smooth.

2. Drape cheesecloth into fine-meshed. Pour in mixture to drain. Tie cheesecloth into a knot. Gently squeeze out liquids. Set aside for 1 day.

3. Place cheese in the fridge for 1 hour to set. Remove cheesecloth. Slice cheese.

Sausage and Cheese Bake

Ingredients:

- ¼ cup uncured sausage, chopped

- ½ tablespoon olive oil

- 1 cup cheddar cheese, shredded

- ½ cup green bell peppers, chopped

- ½ cup red bell peppers, chopped

- 4 eggs, whites only

- ¼ cup lean pork

Directions

1. Preheat the oven to 350 degrees F.

2. Pour water in a skillet. Put sausage and cook for 3 minutes. Set aside.

3. In the same skillet, heat the oil over medium heat. Saute onion and pepper. Add in eggs, cheese, green bell pepper, and red bell pepper. Scatter chopped sausage.

4. Place in a baking dish. Bake for 25 minutes. Serve.

Boiled Sweet Potatoes

Ingredients:

- 8 large sweet potatoes

- water for boiling

Directions:

1. Layer unpeeled sweet potatoes into a large pan set over high heat.

2. Pour just enough water. Bring to a boil.

3. Reduce heat and allow sweet potatoes to simmer for 20 minutes or until tender. Remove from heat. Discard liquids. Serve.

Chestnut Bread

Ingredients:

- coconut oil for greasing

- 2 cups chestnut flour

- $2/3$ cup arrowroot flour

- 3 cups almond meal

- 2 tablespoons coconut flakes, divided

- ½ cup roasted chestnuts, diced

- 1½ teaspoons sea salt

- $2/3$ cup coconut oil

- $2/3$ cup coconut cream

- 2 tablespoons raw organic honey

- 14 large eggs, whites separated

Directions:

1. Preheat oven to 325°F.

2. Line a loaf tin with parchment paper and grease with coconut oil.

3. Combine chestnut flour, arrowroot flour, almond meal, coconut flakes, chestnuts, and se salt. Make a well in the center and pour coconut oil, coconut cream, and honey. Mix until well combined.

4. In another bowl, whisk egg whites until peaks form. Fold into bread batter. Pour batter into loaf tins. Sprinkle coconut flakes.

5. Bake for 40 minutes or until toothpick comes out clean. Allow to cool in tins for 1 hour. Place on a cake rack to cool completely. Serve.

Corn and Raspberry Muffins

Ingredients:

- 1¾ cup whole wheat pastry flour

- 2 teaspoons baking powder

- 1 serving flax egg

- 1⅛ cup coconut milk

- ¼ cup coconut oil

- ½ cup fresh raspberries, rinsed, drained

- ¼ cup canned whole corn kernels, drained

- 3 tablespoons brown sugar

- ½ teaspoon kosher salt

Direction:

1. Preheat oven to 375°F.

2. Place paper liners into muffin tins. Combine flour, baking powder, flax egg, coconut milk, coconut oil, raspberries, corn kernels, brown sugar and salt. Do not over mix.

3. Spoon batter into lined muffin depressions.

4. Bake for 20 minutes or until toothpick comes out clean. Remove from oven. Cool before removing muffins from tins. Allow to cool on cake rack. Serve.

Pistachios Salad

Ingredients:

- 1 tbsp. olive oil

- ½ cup pistachios, unsalted

- 1 cucumber, sliced

- 1 ½ cups cherry tomatoes

- ¼ cup basil, chopped

- 2 cups baby salad greens

- 2 tbsp. sherry vinegar

- Pinch of salt

- Pinch of pepper

Directions:

1. Preheat the oven to 350 degrees F. Grease a baking sheet with olive oil.

2. Spread pistachios in the baking sheet. Place inside the oven and toast for 8 minutes. Set aside.

3. Meanwhile, put together cucumber, tomatoes, basil, and baby salad greens. Season with vinegar, salt, and pepper. Coat well. Add the pistachios. Serve.

Grilled Plantains with Maple Syrup

Ingredients:

- 8 under ripe plantains, quartered lengthwise

- Coconut butter for greasing

- pure maple syrup

Directions:

1. Preheat electric grill.

2. Grease plantain slivers with coconut butter.

3. Grill until brown on both sides. Remove from heat. Drizzle in maple syrup. Serve.

Boiled Plantains

Ingredients:

- 8 large overripe sweet plantains
- water for boiling

Directions:

1. Layer unpeeled plantains into a large pan set over high heat.

2. Pour just enough water. Bring to a boil.

3. Reduce heat and allow plantains to simmer for 20 minutes or until tender. Remove from heat. Discard liquids. Serve.

Plantain Raisins Muffins

Ingredients:

- ¼ cup raisins

- 1½ cups whole wheat pastry flour

- 2 teaspoons baking soda

- ½ cup steel-cut oats

- 2 servings flax eggs

- 4 pieces overripe plantains, mashed

- ½ cup palm sugar, crumbled

- ¼ cup coconut oil

- ¼ cup water

- 1 teaspoon vanilla extract

Directions:

1. Soak raisins in water for 2 hours before using.

2. Preheat the oven to 375°F. Place paper liners into muffin tins. Combine flour, baking soda, oats, flax eggs, plantains, sugar, coconut oil, water, and vanilla extract. Do not over mix.

3. Spoon batter into lined muffin depressions.

4. Bake for 15 minutes or until toothpick inserted in center comes out clean. Remove from oven. Cool muffins before serving.

Spinach Tomatoes in Lettuce Wraps

Ingredients:

- 5 teaspoons extra virgin olive oil

- ½ cup fresh spinach

- 4 large lettuce leaves

- 2 tomatoes

- ¼ teaspoon salt

- ½ cup cheddar cheese

- ¼ teaspoon pepper

Directions:

1. Heat the olive oil in a skillet. Add in spinach. Cook for 3 minutes. Remove from heat and set aside.

2. Top lettuce leaves with spinach and tomatoes. Season with salt and pepper. Serve.

Bacon and Eggs

Ingredients:

- 1 cup water

- ½ teaspoons olive oil

- 2 eggs, beaten

- 2 uncured bacon

Directions:

1. Pour water in a skillet. Bring to a boil. Put bacons and cook for 4 minutes. Set aside.

2. In the same skillet, heat the olive oil over medium heat. Add beaten eggs and cooked bacon. Cook for 2 minutes. Serve.

3. Heat oil in a large skillet and cook the eggs and bacons. Serve.

Breakfast Ricotta Mix

Ingredients:

- ½ cup honey

- ½ cup of Ricotta cheese

- 1 tablespoon maple syrup

- 1 egg

Directions:

1. Using a microwave-safe bowl, combine egg, ricotta cheese, honey, and maple syrup. Mix until all ingredients are well-combined.

2. Microwave for 3 minutes. Serve.

Honey Baked Blueberries

Ingredients:

- 2 cups blueberries

- ½ cup honey

- ½ cup raw walnuts, roughly chopped

- olive oil for greasing

- Pinch of sea salt

Directions:

1. Preheat the oven to 350°F.

2. Line a baking dish with parchment paper and grease with oil.

3. Layer blueberries and sprinkle walnuts. Season with salt. Season with salt.

4. Drizzle honey. Bake for 25 minutes. Remove from heat. Place fruits into individual bowls with nuts.

Rolled Spinach Omelet with Bacon

Ingredients:

- 8 eggs

- 1 cup milk

- 1 cup spinach, cooked

- 1 tablespoon gluten-free mustard

- Pinch of salt

- Pinch of pepper

- 1 cup uncured bacon, chopped

- 1 cup of shredded cheese

Directions:

1. Preheat the oven to 350 degrees F.

2. In a bowl, combine eggs, milk, and spinach.

3. Pour mixture into the baking dish. Scatter cheese and uncured bacon.

4. Bake for 5 minutes.

5. Take out from the baking sheet and roll tightly. Slice into equal pieces. Place inside the refrigerator for 2 hours or overnight.

6. To serve, microwave for 1 minute.

Frozen Yogurt with Fruits

Ingredients:

- 1 tub Greek yogurt, low fat
- 1 cup fresh blueberries
- 1 banana, diced
- 1 peach, diced

Directions:

1. In a bowl, fold blueberries, banana, and peach into yogurt. Mix until well combined. Divide into equal portions.
2. Scoop portions in small containers.
3. Freeze for 5 hours before consuming. Serve.

Sweet Potato Butter with Dried Cranberries

Ingredients:

- 3 tablespoons raw organic honey

- 1 can sweet potato puree

- ⅛ teaspoon apple cider vinegar

- ¼ cup dried cranberries

- Pinch of sea salt

- dash of all spice powder

- dash of cinnamon powder

- dash of cumin powder

- dash of ginger powder

Directions:

1. Process coconut flakes in a blender until smoot

2. Store in airtight container; use as needed.

Turkey Scrambled Eggs

Ingredients:

- Olive oil, for greasing

- ½ cup uncultured turkey slices

- 4 eggs, beaten

- ¼ cup low fat cheddar cheese, shredded

- Pinch of salt

- Pinch of pepper

Directions:

1. Preheat the oven to 350 degrees F. Grease baking dish with olive oil.

2. In a bowl, combine turkey slices, eggs, and cheese. Mix well.

3. Transfer mixture into a baking dish. Top with tomato sauce, turkey slices, and cheese.

4. Place inside the oven and bake for 5 minutes. Serve.

Honey Baked Peaches with Raw Pecans

Ingredients:

- 6 fresh peaches, halved, pitted

- ½ cup honey

- ½ cup raw pecans, roughly chopped

- olive oil for greasing

- Pinch of sea salt

Directions:

1. Preheat the oven to 350°F.

2. Line a baking dish with parchment paper and grease with oil.

3. Layer peaches and sprinkle pecans. Season with salt. Season with salt.

4. Drizzle honey. Bake for 25 minutes. Remove from heat. Place fruits into individual bowls with nuts.

Basil Bruschetta

Ingredients:

- 1 tomato, halved

- 1 Kaiser roll, halved lengthwise

- 1 tablespoon basil pesto sauce

- 1 tablespoon cashew cheese

Directions:

1. On a bread roll, spread pesto sauce and tomato slices. Drizzle cashew cheese on top.

2. Heat the bruschetta in a toaster until warmed through. Serve.

Breakfast Cheesecake

Ingredients:

- 4 eggs

- 7 cups fat free cream cheese

- 7 cups cottage cheese

- 2 tbsp. honey, add more if needed

- 2 tsp. vanilla

- ½ tsp. olive oil

- ½ onion, chopped

- ½ cup uncured sausage

- Pinch of salt

- Pinch of pepper

Directions:

1. In a blender, combine eggs, cream cheese, cottage cheese, honey, and vanilla. Process until all ingredients are well combined.

2. Meanwhile, heat the olive oil in a pan. Saute onion and uncured sausage. Season with salt and pepper. Cook for 4 minutes. Transfer the mixture into a baking dish.

3. Place inside the oven and bake for 10 minutes. Allow to cool at room temperature. Refrigerate for 1 hour before serving.

Crostini with Tomato and Avocado

Ingredients:

- 2 slices wheat bread, toasted

- 2 garlic cloves, peeled

- Pinch of Spanish paprika

For the avocado salad

- 2 tablespoons lemon juice, freshly squeezed

- ½ avocado, minced

- 2 sprigs cilantro, minced

- 1 ripe tomato, minced

- 1 leek, minced

- Pinch of sea salt

- Pinch of white pepper

Directions:

1. Preheat the oven toaster. Rub garlic cloves on both sides of the bread.

2. Meanwhile, combine lemon juice, cilantro, tomato, leek, sea salt, and pepper. Mix and mash. Adjust seasoning.

3. Spread equal portions on bread slices. Place in the oven toaster to warm through. Sprinkle in paprika. Serve.

Watermelon Salad

Ingredients:

- 2 cups salad greens

- 1 cup watermelon, cubed

- 1 tablespoon honey

Directions

1. In a bowl, put together salad greens and watermelon. Toss well to combine.

2. Drizzle in honey.

3. Refrigerate for 1 hour before serving.

Crostini with Capers and Tomatoes

Ingredients:

- 2 slices wheat bread, toasted

- 2 garlic cloves, peeled

- ⅛ teaspoon extra virgin olive oil

For the Vegetable spread

- 1 teaspoon apple cider vinegar

- 1 roasted red pepper in oil, minced

- 1 fresh oregano leaf, minced

- 1 fresh tomato, minced

- 1 teaspoon capers in brine

- Pinch of sea salt

- Pinch of black pepper

Directions:

1. Preheat the oven toaster. Rub garlic cloves on the toasted bread. Set aside.

2. In a small bowl, combine apple cider vinegar, red pepper in oil, oregano, tomato, capers, salt, and pepper. Adjust seasoning.

3. Spread on bread slices. Place in the oven toaster to warm through. Drizzle in oil. Serve.

Frozen Yogurt with Strawberries

Ingredients:

- 1 tub Greek yogurt, low fat

- 1 cup fresh strawberries

- 1 kiwi, diced

- 1 apple, diced

Directions:

1. In a bowl, fold strawberries, kiwi, and apple into yogurt. Mix until well combined. Divide into equal portions.

2. Scoop portions in small containers.

3. Freeze for 5 hours before consuming. Serve.

Baked Chilies

Ingredients:

- ¼ cup almond milk

- 2 eggs

- ¾ cup cheddar cheese, shredded

- 1 can chilies, chopped

Directions:

1. Preheat the oven to 350 degrees F.

2. In a bowl, combine almond milk and egg. Whisk well. Set aside.

3. Put chilies on the baking dish. Pour the milk mixture over the chilies. Sprinkle cheese.

4. Place inside the oven and bake for 30 minutes. Serve.

Creamy Egg Melt

Ingredients:

- 2 eggs, beaten

- Italian seasoning

- 1 cup cheese, shredded

- 1 tbsp. olive oil

Directions:

1. In a small bowl, combine beaten eggs and Italian seasoning. Sprinkle cheese.

2. Heat the olive oil in a pan. Add the egg mixture. Cook for 4 minutes on both sides. Serve.

Bread Sticks with Caraway Seeds

Ingredients:

- 1 tablespoon black caraway seeds

- coconut oil for greasing

For the Bread

- 4 cups almond flour

- 4 tablespoons ghee

- 4 large eggs, whisked

- 1 teaspoon sea salt

Directions:

1. Preheat oven to 350°F.

2. Line baking sheets with aluminum foil. Lightly grease with oil.

3. Combine almond flour, ghee, eggs, and salt in a bowl. Mix until dough comes together.

4. Place dough on lightly floured surface and knead until elastic. Rest dough for 5 minutes, covered.

5. Roll dough and divide into balls. Roll each out into bread sticks and place on baking sheets.

6. Brush ghee on each stick. Sprinkle caraway seeds on top. Bake for 10 minutes.

7. Remove from oven. Let cool and serve.

Frozen Yogurt with Grapes and Melon

Ingredients:

- 1 tub Greek yogurt, low fat

- 1 cup fresh grapes

- 1 cup cranberries

- 1 melon, diced

Directions:

1. In a bowl, fold grapes, cranberries, and melon into yogurt. Mix until well combined. Divide into equal portions.

2. Scoop portions in small containers.

3. Freeze for 5 hours before consuming. Serve.

Chapter 2
Recipes for Lunch

Grilled Beef

Ingredients:

- 2 slices beef

- Pinch of salt

- Pinch of pepper

- Pinch of ground cumin

Directions:

1. Prepare the grill.

2. Season beef slices with salt, pepper, and cumin.

3. Grill for 10 minutes for each side. Serve with bed of greens.

Classic Chicken Salad

Ingredients:

- 1 cup grilled chicken, cubed

- 1 tablespoon white wine

- 2 cups salad greens

- Pinch of salt

- Pinch of pepper

- 1 boiled egg, halved

Directions:

1. In a large bowl, put together grilled chicken, white wine, and salad greens. Season with salt and pepper.

2. Serve with boiled egg on the side.

Pineapple and Watermelon Salad

Ingredients:

- 1 cup pineapple, cubed
- 1 cup watermelon, cubed
- 1 cup salad greens
- Pinch of salt
- Pinch of pepper
- 1 tablespoon honey

Directions:

1. In a bowl, combine pineapple, watermelon, and salad greens. Toss well to combine.
2. Season salad mix with salt and pepper.
3. Finally, drizzle in honey. Refrigerate for 1 hour before serving.

Seared Salmon

Ingredients:

- 1 lb salmon steak, rinsed and blotted dry with paper towels
- 1/8 tsp cayenne pepper
- 1 tsp chili powder
- ½ tsp cumin
- ¾ tsp salt
- 1 tsp freshly ground black pepper
- 2 garlic cloves, minced
- 1 tablespoon olive oil
- 1 lime, sliced into wedges

Directions:

1. Preheat the oven to 350 degrees F.
2. In a bowl, combine cayenne pepper, chili powder, cumin, salt, and black pepper. Set aside.
3. Drizzle in olive oil onto the salmon steak. Rub on both sides.
4. Rub garlic and the prepared spice mixture. Let sit for 10 minutes.
5. After allowing the flavors to meld, prepare an ovenproof skillet.
6. Heat the olive oil. Once hot, sear salmon for 4 minutes on both sides.
7. Transfer skillet inside the oven. Bake for 10 minutes.
8. Serve with lime wedges.

Breaded Artichoke Hearts

Ingredients:

- ½ lemon, sliced into wedges

- coconut oil

- 1 lb fresh artichoke hearts, quartered

- Pinch of sea salt

- Pinch of white pepper

- 1 cup almond flour

- 2 eggs, whisked

- 1 cup almond meal

Directions:

1. In a nonstick skillet set over medium heat, pour oil. Swirl pan to coat.

2. Lightly grease artichokes with salt and pepper. Dredge in almond flour, eggs, and then almond meal.

3. Slide breaded veggies into oil for 1 minute or until crisp and golden. Drain on paper towels. Serve with wedge of lime.

Sweet Turkey

Ingredients:

- 2 turkey breasts
- 2 tablespoons maple syrup
- Pinch of salt
- Pinch of pepper

Directions:

1. Season turkey breast with maple syrup, salt, and pepper.
2. Place the turkey on a greased baking sheet.
3. Bake for at least twenty minutes at 350 degrees Fahrenheit.
4. Serve with salad greens.

Avocado and Crab Salad

Ingredients:

- 2 tablespoons mayonnaise

- Pinch of cayenne pepper

- ¼ cup fresh cilantro, chopped

- 1 tablespoon lime, freshly squeezed

- 1 pound crab meat

- Pinch of salt

- Pinch of pepper

- 1 avocado, cubed

Directions:

1. In a bowl, mix mayonnaise, cayenne pepper, cilantro, and lime juice.

2. Season crab meat with salt and pepper. Dredge in the mayonnaise mixture.

3. Add the avocado slices. Mix well. Serve.

Baked Chicken

Ingredients:

- 2 chicken breasts

- Pinch of salt

- Pinch of pepper

- ¼ cup barbecue sauce, low-sodium, gluten-free

- ¼ cup uncured bacon

- ½ cup green onion, chopped

- 4 plum tomatoes, diced

- ½ cup cheddar cheese, grated

Directions:

1. Preheat the oven to 165 degrees F.

2. Season chicken breast with salt and pepper. Place chicken in a baking dish.

3. Drizzle in barbecue sauce. Top with bacon, onion, tomatoes, and cheese.

4. Place inside the oven and bake for 30 minutes. Serve.

Mango Pear Salsa

Ingredients:

- 1 mango, chunked

- ¼ cup red onion, finely chopped

- 2 pears, cored, chunked

- 1/4 cup yellow bell pepper, finely chopped

- 1/4 cup red bell pepper, finely chopped

- 2 tsp. olive oil

- 3 tbsp. fresh cilantro, chopped

- 1 jalapeño pepper, finely chopped

- Pinch of salt

- 1 tbsp. lime juice

Directions:

1. Mix mango, red onion, pears, yellow bell pepper, red bell pepper, olive oil, cilantro, jalapeño pepper, salt, and lime juice in a bowl. Mix well until all ingredients are well combined. Wrap bowl.

2. Pace inside the refrigerator. Serve as needed.

Mashed Cauliflowers

Ingredients:

- 1 cup cauliflower florets

- 2 tbsp. salted butter

- ¼ cup sour cream

- Pinch of pepper

Directions:

1. Steam cauliflower florets for 5 minutes or until soft.

2. Process steamed florets in a food processor.

3. Add in butter and sour cream. Process again until all ingredients are well combined. Serve.

Salmon Salad

Ingredients:

- 1 can of salmon, drained

- ¼ cup mayonnaise

- 1 cup onion, minced

- 1/3 cup of pickle relish

- 1 celery, minced

- Fresh herbs of choice

Directions:

1. In a salad bowl, put together salmon, mayonnaise, onion, pickle relish, celery, and fresh herbs of choice.

2. Mix all the ingredients until well combined. Serve.

Garlic Pork Chop

Ingredients:

- 3 tablespoons of soy sauce

- Pinch of pepper

- Pinch of salt

- Olive oil

- 2 slices of lean pork chop

- Cumin

- 5 cloves of minced garlic

Directions:

1. In a zip lock bag, combine

2. Place the soy sauce, pepper, salt, pork chops, cumin, and garlic in a zip bag and refrigerate overnight.

3. The next day, heat the oil in a pan and cook the pork chops for three to seven minutes per side or until well done.

4. Serve with fresh fruits.

Greens with Herb Vinaigrette

Ingredients:

- ½ tsp. dried basil

- ½ tsp. dried rosemary

- ½ tsp. dried oregano

- ½ tsp. dried thyme

- 2 garlic cloves, grated

- 1 leek, minced

- 1/8 cup coconut vinegar

- ½ cup olive oil

- 1/8 cup lime juice, freshly squeezed

- Pinch of salt

- Pinch of pepper

- 4 eggs, peeled, preferably soft-boiled

For the Salad

- 1 iceberg lettuce, torn

- ½ cup baby spinach, torn

- ½ cup baby beet tops, torn

Directions:

1. To make the vinaigrette: rub dried basil, rosemary, oregano, and thyme between your palms. Place these herbs along with garlic cloves, leek, coconut vinegar, olive oil, and lime juice. Season with salt and pepper. Shake well.

2. Put iceberg lettuce, baby spinach, and beet tops on a salad bowl. Pour over prepared vinaigrette. Toss well to combine. Spoon into plates and top each plate with an egg. Add more vinaigrette if needed. Serve.

Cajun Shrimp

Ingredients:

- 1 teaspoon of Cajun spice mix

- 1 pound shrimps, peeled

- 2 tablespoons olive oil

Directions:

1. Season shrimps with Cajun spice. Make sure the shrimps are well coated.

2. Meanwhile, heat the olive oil in a skillet set over medium heat.

3. Add shrimps. Cook for 4 minutes or until the coated shrimps turn golden brown.

4. Serve with salad greens.

Baked Sweet Potato Crisps

Ingredients:

- 2 large sweet potatoes, peeled

- olive oil for drizzling

- Dash of Spanish paprika

- Pinch of sea salt

Directions:

1. Preheat the oven to 250°F. Line a baking sheet with aluminum foil.

2. Layer sweet potatoes on baking sheets with spaces in between pieces. Drizzle in oil. Season with paprika and salt. Bake for 1 hours.

3. Cool completely to room temperature. Serve.

Crostini with Smoked Salmon

Ingredients:

- 2 slices wheat bread, toasted
- 2 garlic cloves, peeled
- 4 smoked salmon slivers
- 2 sprigs fresh chives, minced

For the cucumber-capers spread

- 1 tablespoon capers
- ¼ cup tomatoes, minced
- ½ cup cucumbers, minced
- Pinch of sea salt
- Pinch of white pepper
- 2 tablespoon lemon juice, freshly squeezed

Directions:

1. Preheat the oven toaster. Rub garlic cloves on the toasted bread. Set aside.

2. In a small bowl, combine salmon, capers, tomatoes, cucumbers, salt, and pepper. Adjust seasoning.

3. Spread on bread slices. Place in the oven toaster to warm through. Garnish with chives and sprinkle lemon juice. Serve.

Asparagus Bacon

Ingredients:

- 1 tablespoon olive oil

- ½ cup grass-fed bacon, chopped

- 2 cups asparagus, chopped

- ½ cup tomatoes, chopped

- Pinch of salt

- Pinch of pepper

Directions:

1. Heat the oil in a skillet set over medium heat.

2. Cook uncured bacon, asparagus, and tomatoes for 5 minutes or until the vegetables are tender and the bacon cooked through. Season with salt and pepper. Serve.

Cranberry Muffins in Blood Orange

Ingredients:

- 1¾ cup all-purpose flour

- 2 teaspoons baking powder

- 1 serving flax egg

- 1 cup coconut milk

- ¼ cup coconut oil

- 3 tablespoons sweet orange juice, freshly squeeze

- ½ cup fresh cranberries, drained

- ¼ cup shelled walnuts, roughly chopped

- 3 tablespoons palm sugar, crumbled

- ½ teaspoon kosher salt

Directions:

1. Preheat the oven to 375°F.

2. Place paper liners into muffin tins. Combine flour, baking powder, flax egg, coconut milk, coconut oil, sweet orange juice, cranberries, walnuts, sugar, and salt. Do not over mix.

3. Spoon batter into lined muffin depressions.

4. Bake for 20 minutes or until toothpick comes out clean. Remove from oven. Allow to cool before removing muffins from tins. Place on a cake rack. Serve.

Chicken Kale Stew

Ingredients:

- 2 teaspoons olive oil
- ½ onion, chopped
- 2 cloves garlic, minced
- ½ cup mushrooms
- 1 pound chicken, skinless, deboned
- 1 bunch kale
- 1 can tomatoes, diced
- ¼ cup tomato paste
- Pinch of salt
- Pinch of ground pepper

Directions:

1. In a skillet, heat the oil set over medium heat. Sauté onion, garlic, and mushrooms for 3 minutes or until soft.

2. Add in chicken and kale. Cook for 3 minutes or until wilted.

3. Tip in tomatoes and tomato paste. Season with sakt and pepper. Stir well.

4. Allow to simmer for 5 minutes. Serve immediately.

Breaded Baby Spinach

Ingredients:

- ½ lemon, sliced into wedges

- coconut oil

- 1 lb baby spinach, quartered

- Pinch of sea salt

- Pinch of white pepper

- 1 cup almond flour

- 2 eggs, whisked

- 1 cup almond meal

Directions:

1. In a nonstick skillet set over medium heat, pour oil. Swirl pan to coat.

2. Lightly grease artichokes with salt and pepper. Dredge in almond flour, eggs, and then almond meal.

3. Slide breaded veggies into oil for 1 minute or until crisp and golden. Drain on paper towels. Serve with wedge of lime.

Buttered Carrots and Brussels Sprouts

Ingredients:

- 3 tablespoons unsalted butter, divided

- 2 tablespoons onions, chopped

- 1 pound carrots, cut diagonally

- 1 pound Brussels sprouts, halved

- Pinch of salt

- Pinch of pepper

- 1/3 cup water

- 1 tablespoon cider vinegar

Directions:

1. In a skillet, heat the butter and cook the onions until softened.

2. Add the carrots and Brussels sprouts. Cook for 3 minutes or until the vegetables assume a brown color. Season with salt and pepper.

3. Add water. Cover the skillet to allow the vegetables to tenderize.

4. Add apple cider vinegar. Season with salt and pepper. Serve.

Crostini with Mushrooms and Parsley

Ingredients:

- 2 slices wheat bread, toasted

- 2 garlic cloves, peeled

For the toppings:

- 2 tablespoons ghee

- 2 tablespoons olive oil

- 4 porcini mushrooms, thinly sliced

- 1 tablespoon lemon juice, freshly squeezed

- ¼ cup fresh parsley, minced

- Pinch of sea salt

- Pinch of white pepper

Directions:

1. Rub garlic cloves on the toasted bread. Set aside.

2. Meanwhile, in a skillet, pour oil and ghee. Tip in mushrooms for 4 minutes or until golden brown.

3. Pour lemon juice and parsley. Season with salt and pepper. Adjust seasoning.

Aubergine and Courgettes Terrines

Ingredients:

- 1 aubergine, sliced into rounds

- 2 tbsp. extra virgin olive oil

- 2 courgettes, sliced thinly

- 1 fresh thyme sprig

- 4 tomatoes, seeded

- 3 fresh basil leaves, finely sliced

- ½ cup fresh baby spinach

- 1 tbsp. butter

- Pinch of salt

- Pinch of ground pepper

- ½ roasted red pepper, chopped

Directions:

1. Preheat the oven to 190 degrees F. Seal muffin rings with clear film.

2. Meanwhile, heat the olive oil in the skillet. Fry aubergine for 4 minutes or until brown on all sides. Place cooked aubergine on a baking sheet.

3. Cook inside the oven for 10 minutes. Transfer to a plate lined with kitchen paper. Set aside.

4. In the same skillet cook courgettes for 2 minutes. Drain using a kitchen paper. Season with salt and pepper. Sprinkle thyme leaves.

5. Using a heavy-based pan, put oil, tomatoes, and basil. Cook for 5 minutes. Add in butter, garlic, and spinach. Cook until all water evaporates. Stir in nutmeg. Season with salt and pepper.

6. Line the base of muffin rings with spinach leaves. Put courgettes around the edges. Put tomato mixture among the rings. Place aubergines on top.

7. Seal top with film. Chill overnight. Remove from the rings and serve.

Baked Mushrooms and Eggs

Ingredients:

- 3 tbsp. butter

- 2 onions, finely chopped

- 1 garlic clove, finely chopped

- 2 cups wild mushrooms, finely chopped

- 1 tbsp. lemon juice

- 1 tsp. fresh tarragon, chopped

- 2 tbsp. crème fraiche

- 2 tbsp. fresh chives, snipped, reserve some for garnish

- 5 eggs

- Pinch of salt

- Pinch of pepper

Directions:

1. Preheat the oven to 375 degrees F.

2. Meanwhile, Heat the butter in a pan. Cook the onions and garlic for 3 minutes or until browned and softened.

3. Add in mushrooms. Stir frequently until the mushrooms lose its moisture and the color is starting to turn into brown.

4. Tip in tarragon and lemon juice. Put half tablespoon of the crème fraiche and chives. Season with salt and pepper.

5. Distribute mushroom mixture into ramekins. Sprinkle chives.

6. Break an egg into each ramekin. Place inside the oven and bake for 15 minutes or until the eggs are set.

7. Garnish with chives. Serve.

Mixed Vegetables

Ingredients:

- 2 tbsp. olive oil

- 3 turnips, sliced

- 3 leeks, sliced

- 1 red bell pepper, sliced

- ½ cup fresh spinach leaves

- ½ cup artichoke hearts

- 4 tbsp. pumpkin seeds

- Pinch of salt

- Pinch of ground black pepper

Directions:

1. Preheat the oven to 350 degrees F. Pour olive oil unto the casserole.

2. Place leeks, turnips, spinach, artichoke hearts, and red bell pepper in the saucepan.

3. Cover the casserole. Place inside the microwave oven. Bake for 30 minutes or until the turnips have softened.

4. Sprinkle pumpkin seeds. Season with salt and pepper. Serve.

Chapter 3
Recipes for Dinner

Spiced Vegetables with Coconut Milk

Ingredients:

- 2 tbsp. olive oil

- 1 fresh root ginger, grated

- 1 garlic clove, crushed

- 1 fresh red chilli, chopped

- 2 carrots, sliced diagonally

- 4 celery stalks, sliced diagonally

- 2 spring onions, sliced

- 1 can coconut milk

- 1 tbsp. fresh coriander, chopped

- Pinch of salt

- Pinch of pepper

Directions:

1. Heat a wok and pour olive oil. Saute garlic and ginger for 2 minutes or until the garlic is pale golden in color.

2. Add carrots, fennels, chilli, spring onions, and celery. Saute for 2 minutes.

3. Pour in coconut milk. Bring mixture to a boil. Continue stirring until the vegetables are tender and the coconut milk reduces.

4. Season with salt and pepper. Toss in coriander. Serve.

Aubergine Curry

Ingredients:

- 2 tbsp. olive oil

- 2 aubergine

- ½ tsp mustard seeds

- 2 garlic cloves, crushed

- 1 bunch spring onions, finely chopped

- 1 cup mushroom buttons

- ½ tsp. mild chilli powder

- 1 fresh red chili, finely chopped

- 1 tsp. salt

- 1 tsp ground cumin

- 1 tsp. ground coriander

- ¼ tsp ground turmeric

- 1 can chopped tomatoes

- Fresh coriander, for garnish

Directions:

1. Preheat the oven to 400 degrees F.

2. Brush aubergines with olive oil. Prick with fork and place in a roasting tin.

3. Bake aubergines for 30 minutes.

4. Meanwhile, heat the oil in a pan. Fry mustard seeds. Add in garlic, onion, mushrooms, and chillis. Cook for 5 minutes.

5. Season with salt, cumin, coriander, and turmeric. Add tomatoes. Continue stirring and cook for another 5 minutes.

6. Cut baked aubergines in half and scoop flesh. Mash the flesh.

7. Put mashed flesh together with fresh coriander in a pan. Cook for 3 minutes. Serve.

Mushrooms and Fennel Hot-pot

Ingredients:

- 1 ½ cups dried shiitake mushrooms

- 2 tbsp. olive oil

- 2 onions, peeled, left whole

- 1 head of fennel, roughly chopped

- 1 ½ cups button mushrooms, halved

- 2 cups dry cider

- 2 sun dried tomatoes, drained, sliced

- 2 tbsp. sun-dried tomato paste

- 1 bay leaf

- Fresh parsley, chopped, for garnish

Directions:

1. Using a bowl, put mushrooms and pour boiling water. Allow mushrooms to soak for 20 minutes. Drain mushrooms and discard the stalks. Chop caps into small pieces.

2. Meanwhile, heat the olive oil in a large saucepan. Cook the onion and fennel for 8 minutes or until they have softened.

3. Add in button and shiitake mushrooms. Cook for 3 minutes.

4. Stir in sun-dried tomatoes, paste, and dry cider. Put bay leaf. Bring mixture to a boil. Then, reduce to a simmer for 10 minutes.

5. Discard the bay leaf and sprinkle with parsley. Serve.

Button Mushrooms in Creamy Garlic Sauce

Ingredients:

- 1 ½ tbsp. olive oil

- 1 bay leaf

- 2 garlic cloves, chopped

- 2 fresh green chillies, chopped

- 3 cups button mushrooms, halved

- 3 tbsp. vegetable stock

- 1 cup low0fat fromage frais

- 1 tbsp. fresh mint, chopped, reserve some for garnish

- 1 tbsp. fresh coriander, chopped, reserve some for garnish

- 1 tsp. salt

Directions:

1. Heat the oil in a large saucepan. Cook garlic, green chillies, and bay leaf for 1 minute.

2. Pour vegetable stock and add in mushrooms. Cook for 5 minutes or until the stock has been absorbed.

3. Stir in fromage frais, coriander, mint, and salt. Cook for another 2 minutes.

4. Garnish with coriander and mint. Serve.

Apple, Mango, and Radish Salad

Ingredients:

For the salad

- 10 radishes, sliced thinly

- 1 apple, quartered

- 2 celery stalks, thinly sliced

- 1 mango, cut lengthways

- Fresh dill sprigs, for garnish

For the dressing

- 2 tsp. creamed horseradish

- ½ cup low fat crème fraiche

- 1 tbsp. fresh dill, chopped

- Pinch of salt

- Pinch of pepper

Directions:

1. Place sliced radish in a big salad bowl. Add quartered apples, celery, and mango slices.

2. For the dressing, put together creamed horseradish, crème fraiche, and dill in a small bowl. Season with salt and pepper. Transfer to an airtight jug.

3. Drizzle in dressing over the salad. Garnish with dill. Serve.

Orange, Date, and Carrot Salad

Ingredients:

- 1 small lettuce

- 2 carrots, finely grated

- 2/3 cup fresh dates, sliced lengthways

- 2 oranges, segmented

- 2 tbsp. almond, toasted

- 1 tbsp. orange flower water

- 2 tbsp. lemon juice

- 1 tsp. sugar

- ¼ tsp. salt

Directions:

1. On a latter, spread out lettuce leaves. Put the carrots at the center. Surround with dates, oranges, and almonds.

2. For the dressing, combine orange flower water, lemon juice, sugar, and salt. Drizzle in over salad.

3. Put inside the refrigerator before serving.

Curried Mushrooms

Ingredients:

- 2 tbsp. olive oil

- ½ tsp. cumin seeds

- ¼ tsp. black peppercorns

- 3 green cardamom pods

- ¼ tsp. ground turmeric

- 1 onion, finely chopped

- 1 tsp. ground cumin

- 1 tsp. ground coriander

- ½ tsp. garam masala

- 1 fresh green chilli, finely chopped

- 2 garlic cloves, crushed

- 1 fresh root ginger, grated

- 1 can tomatoes, chopped

- ¼ tsp salt

- 4 cups button mushrooms, halved

- Fresh coriander, chopped, for garnish

Directions:

1. In a large saucepan, heat the olive oil set over low heat. Add cardamom pods, cumin seeds, peppercorns, and turmeric. Cook for 3 minutes.

2. Stir in onions, ground coriander, cumin, and garam masala. Cook for 4 minutes.

3. Tip in garlic, ginger, and chili. Continue stirring and cook for 3 minutes. This will, prevent the spices from sticking to the pan.

4. Pour tomatoes. Season with salt and pepper. Let the mixture simmer for 5 minutes.

5. Tip in mushrooms. Cover the pan and allow to simmer for 10 minutes. Discard cardamom pods. Garnish with coriander. Serve.

Sweet Potato and Aubergine Stew

Ingredients:

- 3 tbsp. olive oil, divided

- 1 lb baby aubergines, halved

- ½ cup onions

- 1 tsp. fennel seeds, lightly crushed

- 4 garlic cloves, thinly sliced

- 5 tsp. fresh root ginger, finely chopped

- 2 cups vegetable stock

- 2 lemon grass stalks, finely chopped

- ½ cup fresh coriander, chopped

- 2 kaffir lime leaves, lightly brushed

- 2 small red chillies

- 3 tbsp. Thai green curry paste

- 2 lbs, sweet potatoes, cut into chunks

- 1 2/3 cups coconut milk

- 1 tsp. sugar

- 1 ½ cups mushrooms, thickly sliced

- 1 lime, freshly squeezed

- Pinch of salt

- Pinch of ground black pepper

- Basil leaves, for garnish

Directions:

1. In a pan, heat the olive oil. Cook aubergines for 4 minutes or until lightly browned on all sides. Drain and set aside.

2. Pour the remaining oil. Tip in onion, garlic, ginger, and fennel seeds. Pour the stock, coriander stalks and roots, lemongrass, chillies, and lime leaves. Cover the pan and allow to simmer for 5 minutes over low heat.

3. Put the sweet potatoes and curry paste. Allow mixture to simmer for 10 minutes. Transfer onions and aubergines to the pan. Cook for another 5 minutes.

4. Add in mushrooms, coconut milk, and sugar. Cook for 5 minutes or until the vegetables are cooked.

5. Scatter basil leaves. Serve.

Sunflower Butter Salmon

Ingredients:

- 4 oz salmon fillet

- ½ onion, chopped

- 2 tbsp. olive oil

- 1 tbsp. sunflower seed butter

- ¼ tsp. lemon juice

- ½ cup spinach

Directions:

1. Prepare the grill. Layer salmon fillet on the grill and cook for 5 minutes or until you achieve desired texture.

2. Meanwhile in a skillet, heat the oil. Saute onion for 3 minutes or until the color turns into golden brown. Set aside.

3. In the same skillet, combine sunflower seed butter and lemon juice. Continue stirring for 2 minutes.

4. After grilling the salmon fillets, put them on a bed of spinach. Pour sunflower bitter sauce over the salmon and veggies. Serve.

Grilled Steaks

Ingredients:

- 1 lb steak of any cut, score fat

- 2 tbsp. olive oil

- 2 tbsp. green onion, sliced

- ½ cup lemon juice

- 1 tsp. lemon peel, shredded finely

- 1 tsp. Worcestershire sauce

- 1 tsp. mustard

- 4 tsp. honey

- ½ tsp. salt

- ¼ tsp pepper

Directions:

1. Layer the steak in a baking dish.

2. Meanwhile, in a small bowl, put together olive oil, green onion, lemon juice, lemon peel, Worcestershire sauce, mustard, honey, salt, and pepper. Stir well.

3. Our over mixture over the steak. Refrigerate for 3 hours or overnight.

4. Grill marinated steaks until desired tenderness is achieved. Serve.

Mediterranean Rollups

Ingredients:

- 1 egg

- 1/8 tsp. salt

- 1/8 tsp. pepper

- 2 tbsp. olive oil, divided

- ½ cup sun-dried tomatoes in oil

- 5 kalamata olives, pitted

- 1/8 tsp. parsley flakes

- 1/8 tsp. red chilli flakes

Directions:

1. In a bowl, mix egg, salt, pepper, and olive oil. Whisk mixture until foamy.

2. Heat a skillet. Pour olive oil. Pour the egg mixture, making sure to spread evenly in the pan forming a thin layer.

3. Cook egg for 3 minutes on both sides. Remove and transfer to a plate.

4. Meanwhile, in a food processor, put together tomatoes, olives, parsley, and chilli flakes. Process until the mixture is well blended.

5. Spread mixture on top of the frittata.

6. Roll frittata and cut into bite-sized pieces. Serve.

Vegetable Terrine

Ingredients:

- 1 tbsp. olive oil

- 1 red pepper, quartered

- 1 green pepper, quartered

- 4 fresh green asparagus stalks

- 2 carrots, sliced diagonally

- 1 cup almond milk, unsweetened

- ¼ cup double cream

- 4 eggs, beaten

- ¾ cup full soft cheese

- 1 tbsp. fresh parsley, chopped

- Pinch of salt

- Pinch of ground black pepper

- Salad leaves

- 2 tomatoes, halved

- ½ cucumber, sliced

Directions:

1. Preheat the oven to 350 degrees F. Grease a loaf tin.

2. Put the pepper quarters on a grill rack. Cook for 4 minutes on both sides or until the skins have charred. Transfer to a plate. Cover with kitchen paper. Allow to cool.

3. Meanwhile, in a pan. Pour water. Cook carrots and asparagus for 3 minutes or until tender. Drain with kitchen paper. Peel off skins of pepper.

4. In a bowl, put together eggs, milk, soft cheese, and cream. Stir well. Season with salt and pepper.

5. Arrange vegetables on the loaf tin. Spoon cheese mixture over the veggies. Layer vegetables and cheese mixture and then layer the pepper on top.

6. Cover tin with foil. Pour in boiling water of the roasting tin.

7. Bake for 45 minutes. Remove from the roasting tin and allow to cool. Lift off lining paper. Slice terrine.

8. Serve with salad leaves, tomatoes, and cucumber.

Mushrooms and Baby Onions

Ingredients:

- 2 carrots, peeled, diced
- 2 baby onions, tops and roots trimmed
- 3 tbsp. olive oil
- ½ cup dry white wine
- 1 tsp. coriander seeds, lightly crushed
- 2 bay leaves
- Dash of cayenne pepper
- 1 garlic clove, crushed
- 3 tomatoes, quartered
- Pinch of salt
- Pinch of pepper
- 3 tbsp. fresh parsley, chopped, for garnish

Directions:

1. Heat the olive oil in a pan. Add onions and carrots. Cool for 15 minutes or until the vegetables have turned light brown.

2. Pour white wine. Garlic, coriander seeds, mushrooms, bay leaves, and tomatoes. Cook for 20 minutes or until the vegetables are tender and the sauce thickens.

3. Transfer to a plate. Allow to cool. You may also choose to chill before serving. Drizzle in olive oil. Sprinkle parsley. Serve.

Artichoke Soup

Ingredients:

- 2 tbsp. olive oil
- 1 garlic clove, chopped
- 1 onion, chopped
- 1 celery stick, chopped
- 4 cups vegetable stock
- 1 ½ lbs. artichokes, chopped
- 2 cups almond milk
- Pinch of salt, add more if needed
- Pinch of pepper, add more if needed

Directions:

1. Heat the olive oil in a large saucepan. Saute garlic, onion, and celery. Stir occasionally for 5 minutes.
2. Pour vegetable stock. Season mixture with salt and pepper. Bring mixture to a boil.
3. Reduce the heat. Allow to simmer for 20 minutes or until the artichokes are tender. Let the soup cool before transferring in a blender.
4. Once cooled, process until smooth and creamy.
5. Return soup in the saucepan. Pour milk. Let it simmer for 2 minutes.
6. Ladle into bowls. Adjust taste if needed. Serve.

Vegetables with Cashew Nuts

Ingredients:

- 2 carrots, cut into matchsticks

- 1 red pepper, cut into matchsticks

- 1 green pepper, cut into matchsticks

- 2 courgettes, cut into matchsticks

- Bunch of spring onions, chopped

- 1 tbsp. extra virgin olive oil

- 4 curry leaves

- ½ tsp. white cumin seeds

- 3 red chillies, dried

- 10 cashew nuts

- 1 tsp. salt

- 2 tbsp. lemon juice

- Fresh mint leaves, for garnish

Directions:

1. Heat the olive oil in a pan. Stir fry curry leaves, dried chillies, and cumin seeds for 2 minutes.

2. Add in cashew nuts, carrots, and courgettes. Cook for 4 minutes or until the vegetables are tender.

3. Transfer to a serving dish. Discard dried chillies. Serve.

Salmon with Sweet Potato Puree

Ingredients:

- 3 red sweet potatoes

- 1 tsp. Chinese mustard

- Pinch of salt

- 1 cup balsamic vinegar

- 1 pound Chinese broccoli

- 2 slices uncured bacon

- 4 salmon fillets

- 2 teaspoons yellow mustard seeds

- 2 tablespoons vegetable oil, divided

- 1 ½ tsp gluten-free soy sauce

Directions:

1. Preheat the oven to 400 degrees ᵒF.

2. Prepare sweet potato by wrapping them individually in a foil.

3. In a baking pan, lay the wrapped sweet potatoes and roast for 1 hour. Allow to cool before peeling them.

4. Run peeled sweet potatoes in a blender until smooth. Transfer into a heating bowl.

5. Add mustard. Season with salt. Put inside the refrigerator for 1 hour.

6. Meanwhile, in a saucepan, pour vinegar. Let it boil until reduced. Tip in soy sauce. Remove from heat.

7. In a pot, pour water and salt. Boil the broccoli for 3 minutes or until tender but crisp.

8. In a skillet, cook the uncured bacon until crisp. Drain using paper towels.

9. In a spice mill, process the mustard seeds until it is coarsely ground.

10. Get the fish and season it with salt and pepper. Season it with mustard seeds.

11. In a skillet, heat the oil. Cook the fish, mustard side down. Do so until it is brown but tender in the center. Get the pureed sweet potatoes and reheat it.

12. In another skillet, heat the oil. Sauté broccoli and bacon. Season with salt and pepper.

13. To serve, plate the broccoli, puree, and the fish side by side. Drizzle with balsamic vinegar.

Turkey Salad

Ingredients:

- 1 ½ pounds of sliced turkey breast

- ¾ cups of red grapes

- 4 stalks of celery

- 1/3 cup of pistachio nuts

- Salt

- Pepper

- 1/3 cup of light mayonnaise

Directions:

1. In a bowl, put together turkey, celery, grapes, pistachios, and mayonnaise. Season with salt and pepper.

2. Chill in the refrigerator for 30 minutes. Serve.

Egg Balls

Ingredients:

- 2 hard-boiled eggs, peeled

- 1 anchovy fillet

- 4 kalamata olives, pitted

- 1 tbsp. coconut oil, melted

- 2 tbsp. chia seeds

Directions:

1. In a food processor, combine eggs, anchovy fillet, Kalamata olives, and coconut oil. Process until ingredients are is well-combined.

2. Place inside the refrigerator for 1 hour or until the mixture becomes firm.

3. After 1 hour, shape the mixture into balls.

4. Scatter chia seeds on a plate. Roll balls to coat well. Refrigerate for 1 hour before serving.

Scrambled Shrimps

Ingredients:

- 2 tbsp. olive oil

- 10 pieces of shrimp, peeled

- Pinch of salt

- 3 eggs

- Pinch of pepper

- 1 garlic, minced

- 1 red bell pepper, chopped

Directions:

1. Heat the oil in a saucepan. Saute onion and garlic for 2 minutes.

2. Add in shrimps. Cook for 4 minutes.

3. Crack the eggs on top of the shrimps. Scramble the eggs and cook for another 3 minutes. Serve immediately.

Beef Steak in Balsamic Mix

Ingredients:

- 3 tbsp. balsamic vinegar

- 2 cloves garlic

- 1 tbsp. extra virgin oil

- ½ tsp. dried thyme

- ¾ lb. beef sirloin

Directions:

1. In a zip lock bag put together garlic, balsamic vinegar, dried thyme, and olive oil. Place the beef sirloin. Make sure to massage and beef and are coated well.

2. Refrigerate for 3 hours or overnight.

3. Preheat the grill. Brush steak with olive oil. Grill for 5 minutes on each side. Serve.

Chapter 4
Snacks and Desserts

Apple and Chia Seed Parfait

Ingredients:

- 1 tablespoon cashew nuts, chopped

For the Parfait Base

- 1¼ cups almond milk

- 1 banana, mashed

- ⅛ teaspoon nutmeg powder

- ½ teaspoon cinnamon powder

- 2 tablespoons chia seeds

For the Apple jam

- ¾ cup apple juice, unsweetened

- 2 Fuji apples, diced

- 2 tablespoons chia seeds

- ⅛ teaspoon nutmeg powder

- ¾ teaspoon cinnamon powder

- Pinch of sea salt

Directions:

1. In a bowl, combine almond milk, banana, nutmeg powder, cinnamon powder, and chia seeds. Mix until well combined. Chill in the fridge.

2. Meanwhile, in a saucepan set over medium heat. Combine apple juice, apples, nutmeg powder, cinnamon powder, and salt. Bring to a boil. Allow to simmer for 20 minutes.

3. Turn off the heat. Mash half of the jam using a wooden spoon. Let cool. Set aside.

4. Spoon 2 tablespoons of parfait base and apple jam into parfait glasses. Garnish with cashew nuts. Serve.

Crostini with Olives

Ingredients:

- 2 slices wheat bread, toasted

- 2 garlic cloves, peeled

- ⅛ teaspoon extra virgin olive oil

For the Vegetable Spread

- 1 teaspoon apple cider vinegar

- 1 large black olive in oil, thinly sliced

- 1 roasted red pepper in oil, julienned

- 1 green olive in brine, thinly sliced

- ⅛ cup onion, minced

- ¼ cup cucumber, julienned

- Pinch of sea salt

- Pinch of black pepper

Directions:

1. Preheat the oven toaster. Rub garlic cloves on the toasted bread. Set aside.

2. In a bowl, combine apple cider vinegar, olive in oil, red pepper in oil, olive in brine, onion, cucumber, salt, and pepper. Adjust seasoning.

3. Spread on bread slices. Place in the oven toaster to warm through. Drizzle in olive oil. Serve.

Cinnamon Honey Bananas

Ingredients:

- 1 large banana, chopped into ½ inch

- 2 tsp. honey

- 1 tsp. cinnamon

Directions:

1. In a small bowl, combine honey and cinnamon.

2. Heat the olive oil in a pan. Cook banana slices for 2 minutes or until browned all over.

3. Pour honey and cinnamon mixture over the bananas. Serve.

Banana Cookies

Ingredients:

- 2 ripe bananas, peeled

- 2/3 cup applesauce, unsweetened

- ¼ cup almond milk, unsweetened

- 4 pitted dates

- 1 tablespoon cinnamon

- 2/3 cup coconut flour

- 1 teaspoon vanilla

- 1 1/2 teaspoon lemon juice

- 3 tablespoons dried and chopped cranberries

- 1 teaspoon baking powder

- 2 tablespoons dried and chopped raisins

Directions:

1. Preheat the oven to 350 degrees F.

2. In a food processor, combine almond milk, applesauce, dates, and bananas. Blend until you achieve a smooth consistency.

3. Add in coconut flour, baking powder, cinnamon, vanilla, and lemon juice. Blend for 1 minute. Fold in cranberries and raisins.

4. Pour a baking sheet with the cookie dough. Place inside the oven for 20 minutes.

5. Allow to sit for 5 minutes and let it harden. Serve.

Avocado Pumpkin Seed Parfait

Ingredients:

- 1 tablespoon cashew nuts, chopped

For the Parfait Base

- 1¼ cups almond milk

- 1 banana, mashed

- ⅛ teaspoon nutmeg powder

- ½ teaspoon cinnamon powder

- 2 tablespoons pumpkin seeds

For the Avocado Jam

- 2 avocados, diced

- 2 tablespoons chia seeds

- ⅛ teaspoon nutmeg powder

- ¾ teaspoon cinnamon powder

- Pinch of sea salt

Directions:

1. In a bowl, combine almond milk, banana, nutmeg powder, cinnamon powder, and pumpkin seeds. Mix until well combined. Chill in the fridge.

2. Meanwhile, in a saucepan set over medium heat. Combine avocados, nutmeg powder, cinnamon powder, and salt. Bring to a boil. Allow to simmer for 20 minutes.

3. Turn off the heat. Mash half of the jam using a wooden spoon. Let cool. Set aside.

4. Spoon 2 tablespoons of parfait base and apple jam into parfait glasses. Garnish with cashew nuts. Serve.

Grilled Sweet Potatoes with Pecans

Ingredients:

- coconut butter

- 2 large sweet potatoes, sliced into thick cubes

- 2 tablespoons raw organic honey

- ½ cup pecans, toasted

- Pinch of sea salt

Directions:

1. Preheat electric grill.

2. Grease sweet potatoes slivers with coconut butter.

3. Grill until brown on both sides. Remove from heat. Drizzle in honey, pecans, and salt.

Crostini with Chicken

Ingredients:

- 2 slices wheat bread, toasted

- 2 garlic cloves, peeled

- 2 sprigs fresh chives, minced

For the Chicken-cashew spread

- ½ cup roasted chicken, shredded

- ¼ cup onion, minced

- ½ avocado, mashed

- ⅛ cup celery rib, minced

- ¼ cup cashew nuts, toasted, chopped

- Pinch of sea salt

- Pinch of white pepper

Choco Banana Almonds

Ingredients:

- ½ cup dark chocolate

- 2 bananas, chopped into bite-sized pieces

- Raw almonds, crushed

Directions:

1. Melt the chocolate in a microwave-safe bowl for 1 minute and 30 seconds.

2. Roll chopped bananas on the melted chocolate. Roll over almonds.

3. Refrigerate for 1 hour. Serve.

Chocolate Avocado Pudding

Ingredients:

- 1 ½ avocadoes

- 2 tbsp. chia seeds

- 1 cup almond milk, unsweetened

- 2 tbsp. cocoa powder

- 1 pack whey protein powder

- 4 scoops stevia

- Pinch of salt

Directions:

1. Combine avocadoes, chia seeds, almond milk, cocoa powder, whey protein powder, stevia, and salt in a blender. Blend for 2 minutes or until all ingredients are well-combined

2. Refrigerate for 1 hour. Serve.

Lemon-Blueberry Pudding

Ingredients:

- 3 eggs

- Nonstick cooking spray

- 2 tablespoons maple syrup

- 1 cup blueberry

- 2 teaspoons lemon peel, shredded

- ¼ cup all-purpose flour

- ¼ teaspoon salt

- 3 tablespoons lemon juice

- 1 cup fat-free milk

- 3 tablespoons vegetable spread

Directions:

1. Coat slow cooker with cooking spray. Place the berries and pour maple syrup.

2. Meanwhile, in a bowl, combine maple syrup, lemon peel, flour, and salt. Add lemon juice, milk, and vegetable oil spread. Mix using an electric mixer until well combined. Set aside.

3. In another bowl. Whisk egg whites until soft peaks form. Pour batter over the berries.

4. Cover and cool on high for 2 hours. Cool, uncovered for 1 hour. Serve.

Apple Chips

Ingredients:

- 2 apples, cored, thinly sliced

- Dash of cinnamon

Directions:

1. Preheat the oven to 275 degrees F. Line a cookie sheet with parchment paper.

2. Layer sliced apples in the cookie sheet. Dust with cinnamon.

3. Place inside the oven and bake for 2 hours. Do not forget to flip apple slices every hour.

4. Remove apple chips and let cool. Serve as needed. Leftovers can be stored in an air-tight container.

Crostini with Tapenade

Ingredients:

- 2 slices wheat bread, toasted

- 2 garlic cloves, peeled

- ½ teaspoon extra virgin olive oil

For the Tapenade

- 6 black olives in oil, pitted, minced

- 2 tablespoon golden raisins, soaked in water for 20 minutes

- 1 tablespoon capers in brine, minced

- 1 tablespoon fresh parsley, minced

- 1 tablespoon lime juice, freshly squeezed

- ¼ tablespoon thyme, minced

- Pinch of sea salt

- Pinch of white pepper

Directions:

1. Preheat the oven toaster. Rub garlic cloves on the toasted bread. Set aside.

2. In a small bowl, combine chicken, onion, avocado, celery rib, cashew nuts, salt and pepper. Adjust seasoning.

3. Spread on bread slices. Place in the oven toaster to warm through. Garnish with chives. Serve.

Baked Cinnamon over Apple Raisins

Ingredients:

- 4 apples, cored

- ¼ cup raisins

- ½ cup 100% apple juice

- 1/8 tsp. nutmeg

- 1 tbsp. lemon juice

- ½ tsp. ground cinnamon

- 2 tbsp. brown sugar

- 1 tsp. lemon peel, grated

Directions:

1. Layer apples in a baking dish. Fill them with raisins.

2. Meanwhile, in a small bowl, put together apple juice, nutmeg, lemon juice, ground cinnamon, brown sugar, and lemon peel. Mix ingredients until well-combined.

3. Coat apples with the mixture. Cover with plastic wrap. Set aside.

4. For the remaining cinnamon, place inside the microwave and heat for 4 minutes or until the sauce thickens.

5. Drizzle over apples. Serve.

Honey Baked Apricots

Ingredients:

- olive oil for greasing

- 4 fresh apricots, halved, pitted

- ½ cup walnuts, roughly chopped

- Pinch of sea salt

- ½ cup honey

Directions:

1. Preheat the oven to 350°F.

2. Line a baking dish with parchment paper and grease with oil.

3. Layer apricots and sprinkle walnuts. Season with salt. Season with salt

4. Drizzle honey. Bake for 25 minutes. Remove from heat. Place fruits into individual bowls with nuts.

Grilled Sweet Potatoes with Cashew Nuts

Ingredients:

- coconut butter

- 2 large sweet potatoes, sliced into thick matchsticks

- 1 tablespoon raw organic honey

- ½ cup fresh blackberries

- ¼ cup cashew nuts, chopped

Directions:

1. Preheat electric grill.

2. Grease sweet potatoes slivers with coconut butter.

3. Grill until brown on both sides. Remove from heat. Drizzle in honey, blueberries, and cashew nuts.

Apple Cinnamon Saute

Ingredients:

- 1 tsp. cinnamon

- 1 apple, chopped into bite-sized pieces

- Coconut oil

Directions:

1. Heat the pan. Pour coconut oil. Put the chopped apples.

2. Dab some cinnamon and mix well. Continue mixing for 2 minutes or until the mixture has caramelized. Serve.

Zucchini Chips

Ingredients:

- 4 zucchini, sliced thinly, ends removed

- 2 tbsp. apple cider vinegar

- 2 tbsp. olive oil

- ¼ tsp. salt

- ¼ tsp. ground black pepper

Directions:

1. Preheat the oven to 225 degrees F. Line a baking dish with parchment paper.

2. In a small bowl, pour vinegar, oil, salt, and pepper. Add zucchini. Mix all ingredients until the zucchini slices are well coated.

3. Layer coated zucchini in baking sheets. Place inside the oven. Bake for 2 hours.

4. Remove zucchini chips and let cool. Serve as needed. Leftovers can be stored in an air-tight container.

Crostini with Tomatoes

Ingredients:

- 2 slices wheat bread, toasted

- 2 garlic cloves, peeled

- ⅛ teaspoon extra virgin olive oil

For the Tomato Spread

- 2 teaspoons lemon juice, freshly squeezed

- 1 fresh oregano leaf, julienned

- 1 green tomato, minced

- 1 red tomato, minced

- Pinch of sea salt

- Pinch of white pepper

- Cayenne powder, optional

Directions:

1. Preheat the oven toaster. Rub garlic cloves on the toasted bread. Set aside.

2. In a small bowl, combine chicken, onion, avocado, celery rib, cashew nuts, salt and pepper. Adjust seasoning.

3. Spread on bread slices. Place in the oven toaster to warm through. Garnish with chives. Serve.

Grilled Sweet Potatoes in Coconut Sauce

Ingredients:

- coconut butter

- 2 large sweet potatoes, sliced into thick cubes

- 1 can coconut cream

- 1 tablespoon raw organic honey

- 1 cup fresh blueberries

Directions:

1. Preheat electric grill.

2. Meanwhile, combine coconut cream and honey. Bring to a boil. Stir continuously.

3. Grease sweet potatoes with coconut butter. Grill until brown on both sides. Remove from heat. Drizzle in coconut sauce. Garnish with blueberries. Serve.

Honey Baked Apples with Walnuts

Ingredients:

- olive oil for greasing

- 4 small apples, halved

- ½ cup walnuts, roughly chopped

- Pinch of sea salt

- ½ cup honey

Directions:

1. Preheat the oven to 350°F.

2. Line a baking dish with parchment paper and grease with oil.

3. Layer apples and sprinkle walnuts. Season with salt. Season with salt

4. Drizzle honey. Bake for 25 minutes. Remove from heat. Place fruits into individual bowls with nuts.

Dark Choco Almond Butter

Ingredients:

- ½ tsp. baking soda

- 1 cup almond butter

- 1 egg, large

- ¾ cup sugar

- ½ tsp. salt

- ½ cup dark chocolate, chopped

Directions:

1. Preheat the oven to 350 degrees F. Line a baking sheet.

2. Meanwhile, put together baking soda, almond butter, egg, sugar, and salt. Mix until all ingredients are well-combined.

3. Fold in chocolate. Mix until it forms a dough.

4. Spoon an equal amount of mixture on a baking sheet. Place inside the oven and bake for 10 minutes.

5. Allow cookies to cool before serving.

Spicy Pecan Butter with Chia Seeds

Ingredients:

- 1 cup coconut milk

- 1 tablespoon coconut oil, melted

- 1 can, sweet potato puree

- 3 tablespoons raw organic honey

- 1 cup raw pecans, soaked in water overnight

- 2 tablespoon chia seeds

- 2 vanilla pods, halved lengthwise

- 1½ teaspoon cinnamon powder

- ½ teaspoon ginger powder

- ¼ teaspoon nutmeg powder

- Pinch of salt

Directions:

1. Place coconut milk, coconut oil, sweet potato puree, honey, pecans, chia seeds, vanilla pods, cinnamon powder, ginger powder, nutmeg, and salt into food processor.

2. Process until smooth. Transfer into airtight container. Use as needed.

Chia Seed Bread

Ingredients:

- coconut oil for greasing

- 3 cups almond flour

- 1½ teaspoon baking soda

- $^1/_3$ cup arrowroot powder

- ½ tablespoon chia seed, coarsely ground

- ½ teaspoon sea salt

- ¾ cup coconut cream

- 5 eggs, whisked

- 1½ teaspoons coconut vinegar

- ½ cup butter, melted

- 1 teaspoon chia seeds, whole

Directions:

1. Preheat oven to 350°F.

2. Lightly grease loaf tin with coconut oil.

3. Combine almond flour, baking soda, cup arrowroot powder, ground chia seeds, and salt in a bowl. Make a well in the center. Pour coconut cream, eggs, vinegar, and butter. Stir until well combined. Pour into loaf tin. Sprinkle whole chia seeds on top.

4. Bake for 30 minutes or until toothpick inserted in center comes out clean. Remove from the oven and let cool. Serve.

Crostini with Spinach and Bacon

Ingredients:

- 2 slices wheat bread, toasted
- 2 garlic cloves, peeled

For the Toppings:

- 2 tablespoons water
- 4 streaky bacon
- 1 teaspoon Dijon mustard
- 1 teaspoon apple cider vinegar
- 1 handful baby-spinach leaves
- 1 handful arugula leaves
- Pinch of sea salt
- Pinch of white pepper

Directions:

1. Rub garlic cloves on the toasted bread. Set aside.

2. In a skillet set over high heat, pour water and layer the bacon. Cook until crisp. Place bacon on the bread.

3. Whisk Dijon mustard and apple cider vinegar into the bacon fat. Stir until the dressing blends and emulsifies. Tip in spinach and arugula leaves. Season with salt and pepper.

4. Add equal portions on top of bacon slices. Serve.

Pizza Slice with Spinach Pepper

Ingredients:

- 1 slice pizza loaf, toasted
- 1 tablespoon Basil-Tomato Pesto Sauce
- ½ tablespoon red bell pepper, julienned
- ½ tablespoon onion, julienned
- ½ cup baby spinach
- 1 teaspoon extra virgin oil
- 1 tablespoon Cashew Cheese
- Pinch of salt
- Pinch of black pepper

Directions:

1. Spread basil-tomato pesto sauce on one side of the bread. Layer onions and baby spinach on top.
2. Drizzle olive oil and sprinkle cashew cheese. Season with salt and black pepper. Heat in a toaster oven. Serve.

Stuffed Zucchini Blossoms

Ingredients:

- 10 zucchini blossoms

- 2 tbsp. olive oil

- 2 cups coconut water

- 2 cups coconut flour

- Pinch of teaspoon sea salt

- 1 ½ cups raw cashew nuts

- Water, for soaking

- 3 tbsp. nutritional yeast

- 2 tsp. garlic powder

- ¼ tsp. dried oregano powder

- ¼ tsp. Spanish paprika powder

- 2 tsp. olive oil

- 1 lemon, freshly juiced

Directions:

1. To make the filling, put cashew nuts in bowl filled with water. Let nuts soak overnight. Drain well. Pour cashew nuts, nutritional yeast, garlic powder, dried oregano powder, Spanish paprika powder, olive oil, and lemon in a blender. Process until the mixture is smooth.

2. Spoon an equal amount of filling into the zucchini blossoms. Twist the tips to seal.

3. Pour olive oil into the pan.

4. Meanwhile, combine coconut water, coconut flour, and salt in a bowl. Stir until lumps disappear. Dip stuffed zucchini blossoms. A light coat is fine. Slide stuffed blossoms into the pan and cook for 3 minutes or until golden brown in color.

5. Drain on paper towels. Serve.

Coconut Bread Sticks

Ingredients:

- coconut oil for greasing

- coconut flakes, unsweetened

For the Bread:

- 6 tablespoons coconut flour

- 3 cups almond flour

- 4 large eggs, whisked

- 4 tablespoons ghee

- ½ teaspoon sea salt

Directions:

1. Preheat oven to 350°F/175°C. Line a baking sheet with aluminum foil. Grease with coconut oil.

2. In a bowl, combine coconut flour, almond flour, eggs, ghee, and salt. Mix until dough comes together. Put dough on a floured surface. Knead until the dough is no longer sticky. Let dough rest for 5 minutes, covered.

3. Turn out dough, roll into a log and divide into small balls. Then roll into sticks Roll each out into bread sticks. Place sticks on a baking sheet.

4. Brush each stick with ghee. Sprinkle with coconut flakes on top. Bake for 10 minutes. Remove from the oven and let cool. Serve.

Spicy Cashew Butter with Flaxseeds

Ingredients:

- 1 cup coconut milk

- 1 tablespoon coconut oil, melted

- 1 can sweet potato puree

- 2 tablespoons raw organic honey

- 1 cup raw cashew nuts, soaked in water overnight

- 2 tablespoons flaxseed meal

- 2 large vanilla pods, halved lengthwise

- 1½ teaspoon all spice powder

- ¼ teaspoon nutmeg powder

- ½ teaspoon ginger powder

- Pinch of sea salt

Directions:

1. Place coconut milk, coconut oil, sweet potato puree, honey, cashew nuts, flaxseed meal, vanilla pods, all spice powder, nutmeg, ginger, and salt into food processor.

2. Process until smooth. Transfer into airtight container. Use as needed.

Pizza Slice with Red Bell Pepper

Ingredients:

- 1 slice pizza loaf, toasted

- 1 tablespoon Basil-Tomato Pesto Sauce

- ½ tablespoon red bell pepper, julienned

- ½ tablespoon onion, julienned

- 1 teaspoon extra virgin oil

- 1 tablespoon Cashew Cheese

- Pinch of salt

- Pinch of black pepper

Directions:

1. Spread basil-tomato pesto sauce on one side of the bread. Layer onions and bell pepper on top.

2. Drizzle olive oil and sprinkle cashew cheese. Season with salt and black pepper. Heat in a toaster oven. Serve.

Bruschetta with Tomatoes and Cucumber

Ingredients:

- 1 slice whole wheat bread

- 1½ tablespoons spicy hummus

- ½ tablespoon tomato, diced

- ½ tablespoon cucumber, diced

- ¼ tablespoon chives, minced

- ½ tablespoon pomegranate seeds, lightly drained

- Pinch of kosher salt

- Pinch of white pepper

Directions:

1. Spread hummus on wheat bread. Heat bruschetta in the toaster oven.

2. Meanwhile, in a mixing bowl, combine tomatoes, cucumber, chives, and pomegranate seeds. Season with salt and pepper. Spread on top of bruschetta. Serve.

Spicy Sweet Potato Matchsticks

Ingredients:

- 2 large sweet potatoes, sliced into thick matchsticks

- ⅛ cup honey

- olive oil for drizzling

For the Spice mix:

- ½ teaspoon all spice powder

- 1 teaspoon cinnamon powder

- Dash of ginger powder

- Dash of nutmeg powder

- Pinch of sea salt

- Olive oil for drizzling

Directions:

1. Preheat the oven to 250°F.

2. Line a baking sheet with aluminum foil. In a small bowl, combine all spice powder, cinnamon powder, ginger powder, nutmeg powder, and salt.

3. Layer sweet potatoes on baking sheets. Drizzle in oil. Bake for 1 hour. Remove from heat. Place sweet potatoes into bowl together with the spice mix. Toss well to combine. Serve.

Rosemary Crackers

Ingredients:

- 2 cups almond flour
- ½ tsp. baking powder
- Pinch of salt
- 5 tbsp. Butter, diced
- 2 tbsp. rosemary leaves, chopped
- 1 egg yolk
- 3 tbsp. water
- Almond milk, for glaze
- Rosemary flowers, for garnish

Directions:

1. Preheat the oven to 350 degrees F.
2. In a food processor, combine baking powder, almond flor, and salt. Tip in butter. Process mixture until it resembles breadcrumbs.
3. Add in egg yolk, water, and rosemary. Process again until a firm dough is achieved. Wrap mixture in clear film. Place inside the fridge for 30 minutes to 1 hour.
4. Roll out the dough on a floured surface. Cut out into cracker shapes.
5. Transfer to a baking sheet. Prick with fork. Brush with almond milk. Bake for 10 minutes.
6. Let cool in the wire rack. Sprinkle rosemary flowers. Serve.

Tomato Salad Sandwich

Ingredients:

- 1 slice toasted wheat bread

- 1 tablespoon Red Pepper-Walnut Pesto Sauce

- extra virgin olive oil, for drizzling

- 2 cherry tomato, unripe, quartered

- 2 red cherry tomatoes, quartered

- ¼ teaspoon apple cider vinegar

- ¼ teaspoon balsamic vinegar

- Pinch palm sugar, crumbled

- pinch of kosher salt

- pinch of white pepper

Directions:

1. Spread pesto sauce on one side of the bread. Heat in the toaster oven.

2. Meanwhile, in a bowl, mix together olive oil, cherry tomatoes, apple cider vinegar, balsamic vinegar, sugar, salt, and pepper. Mix well. Spread mixture on bread. Serve.

Honey Baked Strawberries

Ingredients:

- olive oil for greasing

- 2 cups strawberries

- ½ cup walnuts, roughly chopped

- Pinch of sea salt

- ½ cup honey

Directions:

1. Preheat the oven to 350°F.

2. Line a baking dish with parchment paper and grease with oil.

3. Layer strawberries and sprinkle walnuts. Season with salt. Season with salt.

4. Drizzle honey. Bake for 25 minutes. Remove from heat. Place fruits into individual bowls with nuts.

Walnut Cheese

Ingredients:

- 1 cup raw walnuts, soaked in water overnight

- 1 teaspoon lemon juice, freshly squeezed

- ⅛ teaspoon sea salt

- 2 cups water, filtered

- 1 pear, thinly sliced

Directions:

1. In a food processor, combine lemon juice, almonds, and salt. Pour water and process until smooth.

2. Drape cheesecloth into fine-meshed. Pour in mixture to drain. Tie cheesecloth into a knot. Gently squeeze out liquids. Set aside for 1 day.

3. Place cheese in the fridge for 1 hour to set. Remove cheesecloth. Slice cheese.

Carrot Muffin Cake

Ingredients:

- 3 carrots, grated

- 5 pitted dates

- 1 cup lemon butter

- 1 egg

- 1 banana, mashed

- 2 tbsp. melted butter

- 1 tsp. nutmeg

- 1/3 cup almond flour

- Pinch of salt

- 1 tsp. Black strap molasses

- 1 tsp. apple cider vinegar

- ½ tsp. baking soda

Directions:

1. Preheat the oven to 350 degrees F. Line a muffin pan with parchment paper.

2. Meanwhile, in a bowl. Combine egg, butter, banana, dates, nutmeg, and molasses. Stir well until all ingredients are well combined.

3. Tip in almond flour, baking soda, and apple cider vinegar. Mix. Scatter carrots into the mixture.

4. Spoon batter into the prepared muffin pan. Place inside the oven. Bake for 25 minutes. Allow to cool before serving.

Spicy Bruschetta with Spinach

Ingredients:

- 1 slice wheat bread

- 1 tablespoon Red Peppers Pesto Sauce

- 1 teaspoon olive oil

- 1 green tomato, sliced

- 1 cucumber, sliced

- 1 spinach, torn

- Dash dried pepper flakes

- Pinch of kosher salt

- Pinch of white pepper

Directions:

1. Spread pesto sauce on one side of the bread. Heat in the oven toaster.

2. Meanwhile, pour oil in a non-stick skillet set over medium heat. Saute tomatoes.

3. Transfer to a bowl and tip in cucumber and spinach. Season with dried pepper flakes, salt, and pepper. Spread mixture on bruschetta. Serve.

Spinach Chips

Ingredients:

- 20 spinach leaves

- Dash of cinnamon

Directions:

1. Preheat the oven to 275 degrees F. Line a cookie sheet with parchment paper.

2. Layer spinach leaves in the cookie sheet. Dust with cinnamon.

3. Place inside the oven and bake for 2 hours. Do not forget to flip spinach leaves every hour.

4. Remove spinach chips and let cool. Serve as needed. Leftovers can be stored in an air-tight container.

Corn Hummus Sandwich

Ingredients:

- 1 slice whole wheat bread

- 1½ tablespoon hummus

- ½ tablespoon onion, diced

- 1 tablespoon whole corn kernels, canned

- ½ tablespoon green tomato, diced

- 1 tablespoon lime juice, freshly squeezed

- ½ tablespoon cilantro leaves, minced

- ⅛ teaspoon palm sugar, crumbled

- Pinch of sea salt

Directions:

1. Spread hummus on bread. Heat the bread in a toaster oven.

2. Meanwhile, in a mixing bowl, combine onion, corn kernels, tomatoes, lime juice, cilantro, palm sugar, and salt. Spread on top of the sandwich. Serve.

Pomegranate and Avocado Salad

Ingredients:

- ¼ cup pomegranate vinegar

- ½ tsp. cinnamon powder

- ½ cup extra virgin olive oil

- 1 leek, minced

- 1 chilli, minced

- Pinch of salt

- Pinch of pepper

- ½ lb. baby spinach, torn

- 1 avocado, cubed

- 1 lb. iceberg lettuce, torn

- ¼ cup raw cashew nuts

Directions:

1. In a small bowl, combine cinnamon powder, extra virgin olive oil, minced leek, chili, salt, and pepper. Whisk until all ingredients are well combined.

2. Meanwhile, put together baby spinach, avocado, iceberg lettuce, and cashew nuts in a salad bowl. Pour over dressing. Toss well to combine. Serve.

Macadamia Cheese

Ingredients:

- 1 cup raw macadamia nuts, soaked in water overnight

- 1 teaspoon lemon juice, freshly squeezed

- ⅛ teaspoon sea salt

- 2 cups water, filtered

- dried basil leaves, for sprinkling

Directions:

1. In a food processor, combine lemon juice, almonds, and salt. Pour water and process until smooth.

2. Drape cheesecloth into fine-meshed. Pour in mixture to drain. Tie cheesecloth into a knot. Gently squeeze out liquids. Set aside for 1 day.

3. Place cheese in the fridge for 1 hour to set. Remove cheesecloth. Slice cheese.

Grilled Sweet Potatoes with Walnuts

Ingredients:

- coconut butter

- 2 large sweet potatoes, sliced into thick cubes

- 2 tablespoons raw organic honey

- ½ cup walnuts, toasted

- ⅛ cup raisins

- Pinch of sea salt

Directions:

1. Preheat electric grill.

2. Grease sweet potatoes slivers with coconut butter.

3. Grill until brown on both sides. Remove from heat. Drizzle in honey, walnuts, raisins, and salt.

Spicy Cucumber Bruschetta

Ingredients:

- 1 slice wheat bread

- 1 tablespoon Red Peppers Pesto Sauce

- 1 teaspoon olive oil

- 1 green tomato, sliced

- 1 cucumber, sliced

- Dash dried pepper flakes

- Pinch of kosher salt

- Pinch of white pepper

Directions:

1. Spread pesto sauce on one side of the bread. Heat in the oven toaster.

2. Meanwhile, pour oil in a non-stick skillet set over medium heat. Saute tomatoes.

3. Transfer to a bowl and tip in cucumber. Season with dried pepper flakes, salt, and pepper. Spread mixture on bruschetta. Serve.

Raisin Bread

Ingredients:

- ½ cup sultanas

- ½ cup raisins

- 8 tablespoons coconut butter

- 2 teaspoons nutmeg powder

- 1 cup almond flour

- 2 teaspoons baking soda

- 2 teaspoons cinnamon powder

- 2 tablespoons lime juice, fresh squeezed

- 6 pieces eggs, whisked

- 2 teaspoons vanilla extract

- Pinch sea salt

- water for soaking

Directions:

1. Soak raisins and sultanas in water until they double in size. Drain.

2. Preheat the oven to 350°F. Line loaf tin with parchment paper. Grease with coconut butter.

3. In a bowl, combine soaked sultanas and raisins, nutmeg powder, flour, baking soda, cinnamon powder, lime juice, eggs, vanilla extract, and salt. Mix until well combined. Pour batter into loaf tin. Bake for 45 minutes.

4. Remove from the oven and place on a cake rack. Serve.

Chickpea Salad Sandwich

Ingredients:

- 1 slice whole wheat bread

For the chickpea salad

- ½ teaspoon Homemade Tahini

- ¼ cup avocado, mashed

- ¼ cup canned chickpeas, mashed

- ¼ teaspoon fresh parsley, minced

- Pinch of kosher salt

- Pinch of white pepper

Directions:

1. In a mixing bowl, combine tahini, avocado, chickpea, parsley, salt, and pepper. Spread on top of the bread slice.

2. Heat the bruschetta in a toaster until warmed through. Serve.

Sunflower Seed Butter

Ingredients:

- 3 cups raw sunflower seeds

- ¼ cup raw organic honey

- 2 tablespoons coconut oil, melted

- 1 vanilla pod, halved lengthwise

- ½ teaspoon cinnamon powder

- Pinch of sea salt

Directions:

1. Process coconut flakes in a blender until smoot

2. Store in airtight container; use as needed.

Pecan Almond Butter

Ingredients:

- ¾ cup raw pecans, chopped

- 1 cup raw blanched almond slivers

- 1 vanilla pod, halved lengthwise

- 1 tablespoon raw organic honey

- ¼ teaspoon sea salt

Directions:

1. Preheat the oven to 350°F.

2. Line a baking sheet with aluminum foil. Spread nuts on the baking sheet. Bake for 10 minutes or until golden brown.

3. Remove from heat. Cool before placing into food processor. Add vanilla pod, honey, and salt. Process until smooth. Store in airtight container.

Honey Baked Nectarines with Cashew Nuts

Ingredients:

- olive oil for greasing

- 6 fresh nectarines, halved, pitted

- ½ cup raw cashew nuts, roughly chopped

- ½ cup honey

- Pinch of sea salt

- Dash of red pepper flakes

Directions:

1. Preheat the oven to 350°F.

2. Line a baking dish with parchment paper and grease with oil.

3. Layer nectarines and sprinkle cashew nuts. Season with salt. Season with salt.

4. Drizzle honey. Bake for 25 minutes. Remove from heat. Place fruits into individual bowls with nuts.

Coconut-Cashew Butter with Sesame Seeds

Ingredients:

- 2 tablespoons sesame seeds

- 1½ cups raw cashew nuts, halved

- ½ cup coconut flakes, unsweetened

- 1 tablespoon coconut oil

- ¼ teaspoon sea salt

Directions:

1. Preheat the oven to 350°F.

2. Line a baking sheet with aluminum foil. Spread sesame seeds nuts, coconut flakes, and cashew nuts on the baking sheet. Bake for 10 minutes or until golden brown.

3. Remove from heat. Cool before placing into food processor. Pour olive oil and salt. Process until smooth. Store in airtight container.

Spiced Tomato Bruschetta

Ingredients:

- 1 slice wheat bread

- 1 tablespoon Red Peppers Pesto Sauce

- 1 teaspoon olive oil

- 1 green tomato, sliced

- Dash dried pepper flakes

- Pinch of kosher salt

- Pinch of white pepper

Directions:

1. Spread pesto sauce on one side of the bread. Heat in the oven toaster.

2. Meanwhile, pour oil in a non-stick skillet set over medium heat. Saute tomatoes.

3. Transfer to a bowl. Season with dried pepper flakes, salt, and pepper. Spread mixture on bruschetta. Serve.

Coconut Butter

Ingredients:

- 4 cups coconut flakes, unsweetened

Directions:

1. Process coconut flakes in a blender until smoot

2. Store in airtight container; use as needed.

Coconut Butter with Sunflower Seed

Ingredients:

- 2 tablespoons sesame seeds

- 1 tablespoon raw organic honey

- 1 cup sunflower seeds, unsalted

- ¼ cup golden flaxseed meal

- ¼ cup coconut oil, melted

- ¼ teaspoon sea salt

Directions:

1. Process coconut flakes in a blender until smooth.

2. Store in airtight container; use as needed.

Lemon Blueberry Muffins

Ingredients:

- 1½ cup fresh blueberries, rinsed

Dry ingredients

- 1½ teaspoons baking soda

- 2 cups unbleached all-purpose flour

- 2 teaspoons fresh lemon zest

- ½ teaspoons kosher salt

- 1 tablespoon freshly squeezed lemon juice

- 1 cup low-fat milk

- ¾ cup maple syrup

- ⅓ cup coconut oil

Directions:

1. Preheat oven to 375°F.

2. Place paper liners into muffin tins. Combine baking soda, all-purpose flour, lemon zest, and salt. Mix well.

3. In another bowl, combine lemon juice, milk, maple syrup, and oil. Pour wet ingredients over dry ingredients. Stir well.

4. Fold in blueberries. Spoon equal portions into lined muffin depressions.

5. Bake for 25 minutes or until toothpick comes out clean. Remove from oven. Cool muffins. Serve.

Cranberries with Walnuts Muffins

Ingredients:

- 1¾ cup all-purpose flour

- 2 teaspoons baking powder

- 1 serving flax egg

- ¼ cup coconut oil

- 1⅛ cups walnut milk

- ¼ cup shelled walnuts, roughly chopped

- ½ cup fresh cranberries, drained

- 3 tablespoons palm sugar, crumbled

- ½ teaspoon kosher salt

Directions:

1. Preheat oven to 375°F.

2. Place paper liners into muffin tins. Combine flour, baking powder, flax egg, coconut oil, walnut milk, walnuts, cranberries, palm sugar, and salt. Do not over mix.

3. Spoon batter into muffin depressions.

4. Bake for 20 or until toothpick comes out clean. Remove from oven. Allow to cool before removing muffins from tins. Place on a cake rack. Serve.

Nutty Bread

Ingredients:

- 1 tablespoon pine nuts, chopped

- ½ teaspoon sesame seeds

- ½ teaspoon shelled roasted pumpkin seeds

- 1 tablespoon blanched almond slivers

- dash dried basil, shredded

- dash dried thyme, shredded

For the bread loaf

- 4 tablespoons coconut oil

- 1 cup almond flour

- 1 cup coconut flour

- 5 large eggs, whisked

- ¼ cup tapioca flour

- 1 teaspoon baking soda

- 1 tablespoon coconut vinegar

- ¼ teaspoon sea salt

Directions:

1. Preheat the oven to 350°F.

2. Line a loaf tin with aluminum foil. Grease with coconut oil.

3. Combine almond flour, coconut flour, eggs, tapioca flour, baking soda, coconut vinegar, and salt. Pour batter into loaf tin. Sprinkle with pine nuts, sesame seeds, almond slivers, dried basil, and dried thyme.

4. Bake for 30. Remove from heat and let cool for 1 hour. Place in a cake rack to cool completely. Serve.

Coconut and Honey Butter

Ingredients:

- ⅛ teaspoon raw organic honey

- 4 cups coconut flakes, unsweetened

- Pinch of sea salt

Directions:

1. Process honey, coconut flakes, and salt in a blender until smooth

2. Store in airtight container; use as needed.

Upland Cress Open-Faced Sandwich

Ingredients:

- 1 slice pumpernickel bread, toasted

- 1 handful upland cress

- ½ avocado, mashed

- 1 tsp. Colby Jack cheese, grated

- ¼ tsp. balsamic vinegar, for drizzling

Directions:

1. Spread mashed avocado on 1 side of bread. Place upland cress on top.

2. Drizzle balsamic vinegar before sprinkling cheese on top.

3. Heat open-faced sandwich in oven toaster until cheese melts.

4. Cool slightly before slicing. Slice diagonally in half. Serve.

Conclusion

I'd like to thank you and congratulate you for purchasing this book.

I hope this book was able to give you a lot of meal prep recipes that you try and prepare. Meal prepping entails energy and time. It takes a lot of conscious effort from beginning to end. But, once you get into the hang of preparing your own meals, meal prepping becomes easier and would become almost second-nature to you.

The next step is to try and recreate your favorite meals. Share these recipes to your family and friends who are also into meal prepping.

Finally, if you enjoyed this book, please take the time to share your thoughts and post a review on Amazon. It'd be greatly appreciated!

Thank you and good luck!